# *From* UNLIKELY *to* UNLIMITED!

STEPHANIE ANDERSON

# *From* UNLIKELY *to* UNLIMITED!

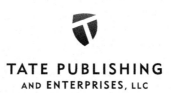

**TATE PUBLISHING**
AND **ENTERPRISES**, LLC

*From Unlikely to Unlimited!*
Copyright © 2016 by Stephanie Anderson. All rights reserved.

No part of this publication may be reproduced, stored in a retrieval system or transmitted in any way by any means, electronic, mechanical, photocopy, recording or otherwise without the prior permission of the author except as provided by USA copyright law.

Scripture quotations marked (NKJV) are taken from the *New King James Version*. Copyright © 1982 by Thomas Nelson, Inc. Used by permission. All rights reserved.

This book is designed to provide accurate and authoritative information with regard to the subject matter covered. This information is given with the understanding that neither the author nor Tate Publishing, LLC is engaged in rendering legal, professional advice. Since the details of your situation are fact dependent, you should additionally seek the services of a competent professional.

The opinions expressed by the author are not necessarily those of Tate Publishing, LLC.

Published by Tate Publishing & Enterprises, LLC
127 E. Trade Center Terrace | Mustang, Oklahoma 73064 USA
1.888.361.9473 | www.tatepublishing.com

Tate Publishing is committed to excellence in the publishing industry. The company reflects the philosophy established by the founders, based on Psalm 68:11,
*"The Lord gave the word and great was the company of those who published it."*

Book design copyright © 2016 by Tate Publishing, LLC. All rights reserved.
*Cover design by Bill Francis Peralta*
*Interior design by Shieldon Alcasid*

Published in the United States of America

ISBN: 978-1-68237-364-4
Health & Fitness / Diseases / Nervous System (incl. Brain)
16.06.13

# CONTENTS

Preface ............................................................. 7

Introduction..................................................... 9

1  From Unlikely Places ............................... 11
2  Unlikely Courage .................................... 17
3  Unlikely Clarity ...................................... 21
4  Unlikely Purpose and Wholeness ........................... 25
5  Unlikely Involvement............................... 29
6  What Is Abnormal Behavior? ................................. 33
7  Unlikely Building Material—Day after Day .......... 37
8  Unlikely Inventory .................................... 41
9  What Is the Strongest, Wisest Influence? .............. 45
10  The Maze of Theory: What Is a Diagnosis? ........... 49
11  Unlocking Your Child's Potential
        Is a Journey Not a Destination ......................... 55
12  Accel-Academy/Conclusion:
        To Unlimited and Beyond ............................... 59

A Debriefing of the Neurodevelopmental Approach ..... 61

## Study and Prayer Guide Quotes, Meditations, Journals, and Prayers

1 From Unlikely Places ................................................. 69
2 Unlikely Courage ...................................................... 73
3 Unlikely Clarity ......................................................... 77
4 Unlikely Purpose and Wholeness ............................ 81
5 Unlikely Involvement ................................................ 85
6 What is Abnormal Behavior? .................................... 89
7 Unlikely Building Material—Day after Day ........... 91
8 Unlikely Inventory .................................................... 95
9 What Is the Strongest, Wisest Influence? ............... 99
10 The Maze of Theory: What Is a Diagnosis? .......... 101
11 Unlocking Your Child's Potential
     Is a Journey Not a Destination ......................... 103
12 Accel-Academy/Conclusion:
     To Unlimited and Beyond .............................. 105

# Preface

In the study of autism treatment, our family found neurodevelopment techniques also termed brain training. I worked with my son from age four to age twelve when our therapy abruptly ended. My husband suffered several strokes and the doctors found a brain tumor.

What I realized as we walked through a very demanding physical and emotional time was that the result of our exercises and brain training with Christian in cognitive, auditory, visual, and tactile areas were permanent. His pupillary response, macular vision and function are typical.

No one who knows Christian today suspects the difficulties he has had to overcome with his diagnosis. I remember thinking he must be a David or Joseph for such a tremendous amount of difficulty to happen at so young an age. Like David, he has written many original compositions and desires to follow his dreams to play music and tell the story of God's miracle in his life. In following his dreams, he wrote a composition for an audition, but had no name yet chosen when he was moments from walking through the door.

He turned to me and said, "How about 'In Good Hands'?" We wrote the title and took the paper to the judges.

Upon our return home, the vehicle slid off the road due to black ice, we flipped several times but our injuries were minor.

There were twelve accidents on the same stretch of road due to the drop in temperature, and we were one of the few families to walk away from the accident.

Christian looked at me as we all walked away from the totaled vehicle and said, "We surely are in good hands."

I am thankful that God intervenes and is directly involved today in our protection. I am also thankful that the brain was created to change with opportunity and heal with proper development.

My son's love for music has given him opportunity to play for veterans, in the community, learn various instruments, write music, lead worship, and play with various projects. It is our dream that many families will find hope and help as we share our story.

May you believe there is hope for every future!

Read more about Christian at
www.hope-future.org/cost-of-a-miracle.html
www.livingworship.wix.com/onesong

To learn more about Christian Michael's music, please visit http://christianmichael.tmgartist.com

# INTRODUCTION

I AM INTRIGUED by the story of *The Woman Who Willed a Miracle*, the true story of a woman, May Lemke, who adopted a six-month-old boy named Leslie who suffered from Cerebral Palsy.

Looking back, I see an unlikely journey that led to miracles when making the decision to parent Christian. The cost of this miracle would be taking a road less traveled and would include hardships, heartache, tears and loss, but would result in strength, peace and hope beyond what I could have imagined.

I made some terrible decisions in my early teens. Some terrifying things happened to me as a young child, which I could not understand or process. I began reaping the consequences of drugs, drinking, and leaving home. But even this was an unlikely opportunity that would allow me to recover what was broken and destroyed. At twenty-six years of age, I admitted I was powerless over addictions, selfishness, dangerous desires, trauma, and hundreds of painful memories. Years later, I would understand and accept that I was powerless in dealing with Christian's lack of function and autism behaviors, and my unknown future was in the hands of God.

In following his dreams, Christian wrote a composition for an audition, but had no name yet chosen when he was moments from walking through the door. He turned to me and said, "How about 'In Good Hands'?" We wrote the title and took the paper to the judges. As we returned home, the vehicle slid off the road due to black ice, and we flipped several times, but our injuries were minor. Christian looked at me as we all walked away from the totaled vehicle and said, "We surely are in good hands." There were twelve accidents on the same stretch of road due to the drop in temperature, and we were one of the few families to walk away from the accident.

I praise God for His remediation and divine intervention. I praise God for the plasticity of the brain and the wonders of His guidance!

Christian's story was posted in the Helena Independent Record.

You can listen to "In Good Hands" through this link: http://youtu.be/roKEpzIviwI. Christian's other biography for talent agencies can be accessed through www.exploretalent.com/christianlane/2325256 with talent number 5684734.

Stephanie Anderson Explore Talent Biography...https://www.exploretalent.com/stephanielane3/2281369

# 1

# FROM UNLIKELY PLACES

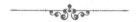

*Yes, the journey is hard, and step-by-step, we will find ourselves in the most unlikely places.*

UNLIKELY IS LIKE a city of chaos where I had dwelt for many years before any of the fragments resembling an undamaged life emerged. As I write and share with you this journey that we have traveled, let me communicate clearly that that there were years between hearing truth in the midst of chaos and what unseen processes were created in moments of hope and belief.

At eighteen months of age, my son began exhibiting violent behavior. He was removed from several daycares to be placed in state programs with testing and evaluations at $300-$600 each time. He was sent to behavioral, occupational and speech therapists. He was shown to have an attachment disorder, oppositional defiant disorder and pervasive developmental delay, a generic autism diagnosis at three years of age.

With each new program, he grew more withdrawn and violent. He still had no cognitive reasoning and few vocabulary words. It was suggested that I send him to an inpatient center for violent toddlers, but when calling advocates for disabled children, I found that state programs/grants wouldn't cover the $2500 a month needed. Another program I found was the Child Behavioral Therapy Unit for extremely autistic children. There was a one year waiting list.

I was told by a caseworker and one of Christian's therapists that a violent toddler's future was normally full institutionalization, so I should consider signing over guardianship of this one I loved so much.

Years later, while providing intervention exercises for my son, I recognized that I was so much like him. I did not accept, agree or cooperate with opportunities or guidance that was meant for my good. Oppositional defiance was somewhat part of my nature as well. Hearing a truth or promise is one baby step; there was no promise or hope in what I was hearing. Thankfully there were moments where I couldn't and wouldn't believe there wasn't an answer.

Most of the first years of recovery after trauma, addictions or abuse begins with passive and consistent input into our hearts and lives after hope and health have been destroyed. How I perceive them depends on my own story, circumstances, failures, or successes—and these are footsteps in unlikely places.

When I first heard Linda Kane talk about the issues some of the families and children she served were facing, I realized I was not alone. *That moment* began change in my life.

My life quote is this: "I know the plans I have for you, plans to prosper you and not to harm you. Plans to give you hope and a future." I read this during a season in my life where I was beginning to see delays and difficulties that appeared permanent.

Maybe you are in a place right now where hope has fled and there is no vision for what is up ahead. I was in that place—a most unlikely circumstance encountering severe problems with Christian's tactility, speech, and vision. Desperation can be the doorway to unlikely creativity and courage.

I was told by one of the counselors at the child development center that I was Christian's only advocate. There are facts, and there is truth. The truth is that the God who formed Christian and watched over him in my womb was just as involved in forming Christian's heart, life, and future here and now in this most unlikely place as He was when He first formed his tiny hands, feet, and nervous system. I had a choice to believe the functions I saw or the promise of God.

A family raising a child with disabilities can be defined as *captive*. From the moment of waking to the sometimes-remote hours of sleeping or sleeplessness, it feels like we don't have a right to the hours, schedule, or any area of own lives.

Desperation marks many of the hours dealing with screaming, with a child who bangs, or during the many trips to the hospital for the child who can't feel pain and hurts himself seriously. The entire family is captive. When we started, a change in schedule would result in screaming for hours with rigidity in muscles, making him too heavy to carry, biting, throwing, scratching, punching, and kicking. Change was an unknown trigger.

The source of behaviors common to children and adults are misunderstood and so are the labels attached to them. According to M & L Special Needs Planning, 20.9 million families have members with a disability.

From before birth in the womb to the continued explosive growth of the brain and stages of development that happen with passive, normal experiences in life, each brain and nervous system goes through certain stages, similar to points toward a destination on a map. These are not forced but very natural processes that God has instinctively patterned in human beings. Sometimes development is interrupted, which can happen because of abuse, trauma, sin, injury, sickness, or a variety of environmental causes, resulting in a very different journey towards achieving their potential and purpose.

One of the most difficult steps in this journey is what is revealed when our expectation or plans are suddenly changed. A parent may see this like having bought a ticket to travel to New York, but they suddenly exit to see a strange culture and destination—requiring knowledge very different than what they had prepared for of a language, map and future.

Because this isn't in our control, we have the process of discovering, rather than planning the years ahead. If the unknown has released overwhelming fear, anger, and tears, you are not alone. This unlikely unknown can be the defining moment for belief, courage, and healing. God is very close to us during every moment, every step.

> **You may not be able to see all the stars in a constellation at this moment in time. Remember— this is only one moment, out of focus and colored by difficulty.**

# 2

# Unlikely Courage

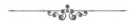

*We tend to separate our mind, will, and emotions
from our physical experience, but there is a link
between what happens in this world and how
it affects the unseen and the eternal.*

IN OUR JOURNEY, there are opportunities for the development of courage. Potential exists for growth in every situation, and the way we interact with those situations is through physical sense and emotion.

A child crawls on his belly, then creeps on his knees, sits/stands, and walks in cross pattern in natural progression without coercion. There are nerve connections being formed in millions of unseen pathways during this process. When a child moves from crawling on the belly to creeping on the knees, the child's visual system is given opportunity to develop depth perception and to see a fixed point in space that will bring macular vision and create a foundation for reading later on.

All physical functions begin in the brain and central nervous system. The sensory nerve systems are bringing information through light, colors, sounds, speech, textures, colors, and smells that give the brain opportunities to respond or learn to filter—loud or soft, far or near, tickle or pain (light and deep pressure sensors) and will organize this information every day.

In the science and research of the development of the brain, a neurodevelopment rehabilitation team worked with brain-injured children, noting that injury to different areas of the brain would result in specific distorted behavior or function. In surgery and treatment for stroke patients, they began to provide exercises to the damaged area of the brain with specific stimulation and found that the brain had plasticity and would begin seeking out new pathways for the incoming sensory opportunities. Individuals regained speech, vision, balance, hearing, and a number of functions after a period of time—some sooner, some months to years later depending on the level of injury.

When we see and hear physical breakthroughs described, we are shown that we have a God who can begin the process of healing or rehabilitation at any time. Creating the opportunity at the specific level we need at the precise time for the proper length at the right intensity is another aspect of God's ability to meet us right where we are.

**The miracle of the brain is its ability to respond to new stimulation.**

**Healing can begin at any moment.**

In the physical realm, we now know that specific functions and behaviors are controlled by specific areas of the brain. If you ask a neurosurgeon, they will tell you the specific functions that could definitely be affected by a tumor or lesion. Every area is different in how a cut, even with precision, can affect millions of cells.

There are many things that can affect our soul and spirit that will affect our life similar such as a tear affecting an area in the brain. Most things in the universe are too small or move too fast or even too slow for us to see.

One night, as Christian slept, I began weeping thinking about the words of the caseworker. Institutionalization? Signing over guardianship? Tears came quietly but constantly.

I opened by Bible. I believed in my heart that if God had given me this child, then He would give me everything I needed, even the strength to let him go if that was best.

My thoughts and memories from the past were like a cloud in my mind. "Maybe I deserve to lose him—I have made such a mess of my life."

I looked to the open Bible. John chapter 9 was where I glanced and began reading. "And His disciples asked Him, saying, 'Rabbi, who sinned, this man or his parents that he should be born blind?' Jesus answered, "Neither this man nor his parents sinned," said Jesus, "but this happened so that the work of God might be displayed in his life..." (New International Version John 9:1-3).

As I read this through my tears, an unexplainable peace came over me. In my heart I had believed that this situation was my deserved punishment because of the mistakes and sins of my life. But in that moment, something had changed forever. I no longer believed I was being punished at all. Somehow this would bring hope to others and glory to God.

> **When we define success for ourselves, we cannot forget the unseen spiritual reality that is developing in us, through us, and around us.**

# 3

# UNLIKELY CLARITY

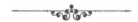

> How one views the nature of God impacts how
> one views anything that occurs in his world.

THERE IS A maze of distractions, influences, and therapies that can lead toward or away from truly helping ourselves and our children. There are influences in the education, medical, and therapeutic communities constantly stating that restoration is unlikely.

I was thankful for any intervention. I received a call from the Child Behavioral Therapy Unit, who had been informed about my desperate situation as a single mother, and would accept Christian into their program. The charge for this four hour program was $110.00 each day.

The September 1999 report (appendix) reads, "Christian had 54 physical aggressions to persons, (hurting himself, throwing himself off things) 19 physical aggressions towards object, (throwing toys, chairs) and 9 bites to others." He had been in attendance for fifteen days.

At the time I conceived Christian, I had little understanding of physiological development or the brain. Developmental issues such as hearing too much of certain tones, not feeling pressure or pain appropriately will show up in unusual behaviors, which are often misunderstood. It is important that opportunities for development are intentionally created. The potential of every child—physical, academic, emotional, and spiritual—hangs in the balance.

Christian Michael was known by the doctors at Holy Cross Hospital in Salt Lake City, Utah, as Bubba. He was a healthy ten-pound, six-ounce baby boy. The labor had been exhausting, and he had been in the birth canal for a prolonged period of time. They finally called in a team of specialists to assist, and an emergency C-section was mentioned. Silently I prayed, "Please don't let that happen, Lord."

Christian emerged with the next push—just a tiny, bruised, very purple creature, but sounding very healthy. I held him and couldn't believe he was finally here. His father and I stared at the tiny hand that was grabbing my finger so tightly. That was one of the few perfectly peaceful times his father John and I had ever spent together. My heart truly believed in that moment, our lives could be different, even good.

John hadn't held a steady job, so I had worked and saved up for the meantime. Now that our savings was used up, I needed to go back to work. Being Mr. Mom seemed to fit John at first, but he began to grow restless, more irritable, and then violent.

I happened to come home a couple of times when he had the music up deafeningly loud and Christian was asleep as if nothing was happening. After checking on him and finding him to be breathing and responding okay, I formed the conclusion that he had adjusted to the noise level. But what I didn't know at the time was Christian's auditory system had been seriously affected.

Christian began having tantrums where we could not comfort him. I found only two things that helped (with the advice of a counselor). If I could get him into the car seat, I would put in ear plugs and drive until he screamed himself to sleep. The other began with a battle for bedtime. I left him in his crib and went for a walk around the block or down the road. I would return quietly so that he would not know I was home. The measure was hard at first because he would scream for a couple of hours at first and start up again if he heard a sound. But within a couple of weeks, he started to fall sleep on his own.

John's attitude was also changing. He began to leave as soon as I walked in the door, and then he stopped coming home until early in the morning. Soon he wasn't coming home at night, and his temper and outbursts were often explosive. When he confessed to being in love with someone else, we separated.

I called a church during this time, and they started meeting with me, praying and fasting for my son and I. They taught me that the Bible was God's word, which has more truth and holds more weight than circumstances. I realized I had many wrong beliefs—I was convinced I knew God—but I knew him no better than Elizabeth knew Mr. Wickham in Pride and Prejudice. God loved me and knew of my dire situation long before I arrived at this point in time. He sent His Son Jesus to die on the cross—to provide redemption that would reach through time and space and release power now and here so unmistakeable that I would never doubt His love or forget His faithfulness. I would learn what was essential for life and faith in the desperation of becoming a single parent.

In the midst of seeming captivity, we don't always understand the reason for situations but this moment know there is a choice. We can trust God.

# 4

# Unlikely Purpose and Wholeness

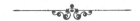

Every child can reach his or her purpose in God.

We know the brain and central nervous system develop through natural stages, unless there is an abnormal, observable behavior present to let us know there is a problem.

There are many types of delays and injuries controlled by millions of nerve pathways that control different behaviors and functions in the brain. We notice lack of function immediately in children with the Down's syndrome look or notice immediately when a child is stemming or exhibiting autistic behaviors. Mild visual function impairment is difficult to detect but easily labeled with reading problems, auditory processing difficulties, and delayed speech. Perceptual problems cause a child to have difficulty in taking in the world through his senses. He may be getting too much sensation or too little.

A child's life is more than the snapshot examinations, testing, and especially labels. Change can begin at any moment, and a child's function is part of a huge tapestry that we only see pieces of. We need to know what our children can do, what level they are processing and create an environment with intentional opportunities for development.

There are underlying nerve brain inputs, outputs, and function that we can observe. At a typical level of development for a newborn, children should have reflexive response to sound, light, and touch. As the child grows, he or she develops feeling sensation (light and deep pressure), tonal processing through filtering sounds, and recognition of faces. The child will begin to grasp, roll, army crawl, creep, and develop the visual system and depth perception and macular vision many months before they will actually perform reading. Eventually the child will stand, walk cross pattern, hear, and understand and respond to conversations. They are gathering all that is needed for life through their senses, experiencing every cool breeze, warm water, firm floor, soft shirt, music, speech, attitude, and tone in their surroundings. Input equals opportunity, and development is the result.

Just as many unseen processes happen in physical development, we do not see the very beginning stages of our relationship with God. Reflexes are being developed as we learn to read and listen to that which creates faith, hope, and knowledge to make wise choices. Everything that we receive is gathered, processed, and filtered through this life, but affects us far beyond this life. We have opportunity for development with input choices: books, movies, music, service, and relationships can help or hinder our development, similar to a baby receiving sensory or nutrient "input" that helps or hinders development.

I had much to reflect on during this time and began the process of taking inventory of my life and actions. I began admitting to myself and God the wrongs I had committed. I also made a list of those who had hurt, abused and betrayed me. I came to understand that forgiveness didn't mean that I would accept any more abuse or injustice from them, but I needed to release my resentments. I chose to forgive.

I wrote letters and began the process of making amends where it was possible. I realized that my focus was turning from myself to caring for others and I found peace and joy in the midst—another hidden treasure from choosing this road less traveled.

# 5

# Unlikely Involvement

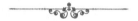

*Similar to a military landing on an occupied island, there is chaos when God steps in.*

In spite of our efforts, errors, and attempts, which so often oppose God, He quietly and consistently begins the work of showing us His faithfulness, over and over; silently, progressively, and carefully acting on our behalf. I believe He rejoices every moment that we respond or even glimpse that He is the one responsible.

In my shattered life, the pieces were beginning to be restored to God's original design. Parenting is an abstract art where imperfect people have the opportunity to discover that God's way is best.

God has an order for every home. It is not a casual occurrence or accident. That means time and attention are spent consciously. Activities aren't necessarily religious, but the atmosphere and events of life are ordered in the understanding that we choose how we spend the 86,400 seconds we have been given each day. Just as what we put in our mouths will affect physical development, how we spend our time will affect the physiological, spiritual, and emotional development our children.

When I looked into Christian's tiny face and beautiful, curious hazel eyes, I knew how much I loved him but also knew that God's plan for his life was the most important of all. In order to fulfill that purpose, we would have to find a way through the terrific challenges that were ahead.

For the single parent, there are few hours that we are allotted to spend with our children that caused me to look at how I spent and valued time—which I did not have an appreciation of before—and every resource. I knew that I was responsible for the healthy physical development of Christian's visual, auditory, and sensory systems, and he needed spiritual and moral development as well.

I didn't want to waste the few hours that I had. I had learned not being able to afford a phone, that it was a luxury, not a necessity. So our time in the evening was sacred. There was no television, and later, when I could afford a phone, the ringer was off. After visits to the park we would eat dinner, listen to Christian radio, play on the floor, bathe, sing songs, pray, and then it was bedtime.

One of the biggest problems I was informed of was Christian's difficulty with transitions. From one activity to the next, there could result an explosive tantrum. This could occur at leaving him, picking him up, or during the break from one therapist to the next at the behavioral program. This is similar to the stroke patient who suddenly needs a sense of sameness and becomes angry when his personal items are moved or schedules are changed. The brain tries to create order internally by controlling the order of the environment externally. I didn't find that to be the case at home because we kept a routine schedule that rarely changed. We didn't do very many social activities, and Christian did very well with me one-on-one with few outbursts. He responded well in a quiet environment, to firm and consistent discipline.

Without God's intervention, the words of doctors would have indicated Christian would have no self-control so no discipline; there would be medication and institutionalization.

I am thankful for having a paradigm of the nature of God versus the nature of man. Christian and I were human beings with sinful hearts. I knew that all persons, including children, were born with a bias toward evil. I also knew that if any child was left to himself, he would be certain to choose wrong because we have an enemy that is far more adept at deceiving, with hundreds of years of experience over ours.

I cried out for wisdom, knowing that I had been making the wrong decisions for most of my life, and in order to persevere, I would require much molding of my own character. I needed to know God's wisdom if I would ever be successful in guiding Christian's heart, mind, and character in the years to come.

# 6

# WHAT IS ABNORMAL BEHAVIOR?

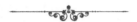

Truth and wisdom are what exists after man's opinions disappear.

STUDYING HISTORY WILL show you how the opinions of life and beliefs of individuals such as Hitler affected him and hundreds of other people. Those supporting Hitler had opinions but little truth to base their opinions on. The special needs community of children and adults were treated as little more than lab rats and destroyed by those who placed no value on their souls. What we believe and why matters.

We see children who can walk but not talk as disabled. There are children and adults who can't talk or understand spoken words and can't be left alone for ten seconds because of various wild behaviors. There are children and adults with such hyperactivity that they are unable to do anything that would be considered human. Those who have operated on injured brains know that if a person wakes up from surgery with any of these severe behavior problems, they have a moderate brain injury.

Behavior is such an important area to understand. There are those who use drugs, conditioning, and psychiatry to address behaviors, addictions, and pain. From mild emotional distress/depression to severe rage and psychosis, unlocking the mystery of behaviors affects the paradigms of cultures and countries. Autism has been a mystery and is one of the most baffling and extreme of the behavioral disorders because there are so many unique points on a spectrum for each individual.

When Christian turned eighteen months of age he began exhibiting extreme and violent behavior. He was removed from several daycare centers because he was hurting other children and teachers. I learned how to distract Christian in the midst of his tantrums with a bag of fun objects that would stop him from cycling into rage. I could see when his little face was growing red and hear when the cry was changing pitch. Sometimes I would blow up a balloon and let the air out quickly in front of him. Sometimes I would blow a quiet whistle. I had bells, colorful rings, stuffed animals, and we never left home without the "alarm" bag.

What wasn't known by the daycare center workers and teachers was the final episode of John's rage that we had endured and survived. For several months we would only see John from time to time when he came to time to visit Christian. On this occasion, I was living in my parent's basement, when John came on an unannounced visit. He fell into such a deep sleep that I could not wake him. I suspected he had been doing drugs; his complexion, dilated eyes, and demeanor added up. I searched his bags and found a gun and hid the bag.

John woke up angry and started calling me names, cursing, and pulled the phone out of the wall. I prayed and quietly picked up my Bible as he ranted. As he became more explosive, I began reading Bible passages out loud. He began picking items off the table and throwing them at me, anything he could get his hands on. Christian was standing behind me as I continued to speak the Word of God out loud. I noticed the objects John was aiming at me never hit either Christian or me. John's body became rigid, and suddenly he came walking toward me screaming, "I will kill you, shut up!" I felt his hands around my head, and I saw him head butt me, but I barely felt it. I had closed my eyes, and slowly I opened them. John was at my feet, crying softly, and quietly said, "I wish I had your faith."

I told him, "Someday you will, now go to sleep."

As he walked to the bedroom, I wept and thanked God for keeping us safe. I took Christian in my arms, and he fell asleep, and I laid him down. I turned on the radio to hear the verse of a song: "Until you are saved, I will pray for you." I began sobbing as I stood there. I wanted to curl up into a little ball on the floor but felt a force that was like arms holding me up as I just cried and leaned on God in a way I had never known I could.

# 7

# Unlikely Building Material—Day after Day

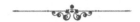

> Practical day-to-day activities are part of the
> journey, part of learning about faith.

When Christian was younger, I volunteered to teach Sunday school. At first he loved the nursery and toys, and it was only one Sunday a month. But Christian's aggression and lack of verbal communication caused problems. He seriously bit or hurt children each week. I tried to take him with me to my class, but soon he was lashing out, and I was losing control of the other kids and having to hold mine in restraint. By the second month, I was staying and serving in the nursery with him, but when the lashing out was turning on me, I stepped back from church attendance.

It was also a difficult time for any socialization in public places. The first was the ball pit at the local fast-food restaurant. I had been meeting with other single moms each month for fellowship from a support group at the local crisis pregnancy center. I can remember the screams and having to climb up into the pit and separate Christian from the arm of another child who was bleeding. Two other visits had similar results, and I stopped visiting indoor playgrounds unless we were the only ones there. Outdoor playgrounds seemed less of a threat where I could watch him every moment. I knew when he was getting ready to strike, and it was at a perceived distance from five to ten feet.

Christian began attending a new program at the Child Behavior Therapy Unit (CBTU) in September of 1999. The ratio was two students to one adult. There were seven students in each class with their individual programs, goals, and challenges. These were all high-functioning, autistic-labeled children with behavioral issues of different sorts. The program required parents to participate twice a week in the classroom while their child was in the program, so I was able to learn and see progress of the students.

I was told that one of the students stuck a key in the electric socket. When it appeared to explode, he didn't react and even seemed oblivious to the burn marks on his hands. I know now that if the boy was feeling pain appropriately, he would have reacted in some way.

When I looked at the first report of attendance, my mother's denial and protective mask was gone. I had been told by good-meaning people that he would grow out of the behaviors. The fact was Christian had fifty-four physical aggressions to persons, nineteen physical aggressions toward objects, and nine bites to others in the first fifteen days. (See appendix.)

Christian spent six months at the CBTU program and then was removed as we relocated to Southern Utah in March of 1999. That summer, I attended a conference where I met Linda Kane, of Hope and a Future. She was an ICAN neurodevelopmentalist that approached developmental delays and labels in a very different way than any other therapist we had visited with. She talked about children being created in the image of God and that each stage of development in a baby's life is important to avoid function problems later on.

Today, I know that keen observations give many clues as to what each child is dealing with. Types and levels of noise they can tolerate (auditory system) or tones they don't say or process; lights and colors (visual system); order and sameness (spatial); textures and pressure upon the skin (tactile system); tastes, odors, and textures (olfactory system). Christian hated loud noises, and even the vacuum would cause him to put his hands over his ears. His auditory system was taking in more than what was typical, and there were sounds that hurt him.

Linda Kane described how each one of Christian's function issues could be addressed with exercises. Growth and development were only a matter of time and opportunity. I took every article she had printed at the table and started immediately. Later we used sound therapy to normalize how he heard tones and sounds. My prayers were being answered.

# 8

# Unlikely Inventory

*The brain stores information, not like a photo
album that can be closed at will, but more like
an open gallery that places photographs
in moments by association.*

THE MOST DIFFICULT reading I did in my research was in regard to the myths and superstitions that clouded entire civilizations in the understanding of the causes of children's problems. One of the false prophets pointed to the cause for autism as refrigerator parents—aloofness of parents and lack of warmth to children caused psychosis that affected behaviors and learning. The filter of theories through which children were being seen was totally clouded. Many psychotherapists religiously confer the source of psychotic and sensory issues seen with disorders like autism upon their parents.

Daycare workers, specialists, and teachers who dealt with Christian made many suggestions based on this theory. The three Ds were present—a father who did *d*rugs, *d*ivorce, and lack of *d*iscipline. Only after Christian was evaluated by professionals, did I stop blaming myself. And every time I thought of how much I had been forgiven, I could give grace and forgiveness to others who didn't know that Christian had far worse issues going on.

A special inventory of our past, our history, and our present can reveal places in our thinking where we hold ourselves, other people, places, or situations responsible. Whether we have had a list that is lines long or pages long, we can ask the Lord to reveal to us what memories "snapshots" are hanging in our minds.

For those that have received forgiveness and salvation through Jesus Christ, the cross is the power of God. We experience so much in the emotional and experiential areas of life: trauma, abuse, neglect, and fearful circumstances and patterns repeated because of issues in relationships. Anger terrifying memories, abuse, and unforgiveness can cause delays in healthy emotional development. Every one of us stores in the brain every image seen, heard, and felt, but God has given us a filtering and storage system for the millions of images from life (subconscious), like a file cabinet. We can push down emotions, we can try creative visualization, but it does not erase; only displacement occurs until we make the association again. If you watched "My Fair Lady," you can remember when an association bypassed her training and she reverted to speech she had carefully disguised.

We do not have to keep focusing on painful and traumatic images with His help. The power of God to heal is necessary before we can truly pray for peace to reign right where we are. Forgiveness accesses that power, and it is possible the moment we act in obedience rather than feelings or rights.

Corrie Ten Boom and her family helped save an estimated eight hundred lives while protecting Jews from arrest by Nazi authorities during World War II. Her entire family was incarcerated for their efforts. Corrie's eighty-four-year-old father died shortly after the arrest, and her sister died during their stay at the notorious Ravensbruck concentration camp.

Corrie was released one week before all the women her age were killed. She once described speaking before a congregation in Munich about her experiences. A particular guard from Ravensbruck, who had watched them stripped of clothing and possessions, who had supervised the humiliation and abuse that eventually took the life of her sister, was sitting in the back of the room. As the meeting ended, he began to walk up the aisle. She described the intense hatred that surfaced with horrific memories still trapped in her memory. She froze with anger and repulsion for this man. But the One-Who-Forgives, who is greater in us, gave her the strength as she silently warred, prayed, and asked for the means to forgive. She states that as he extended his hand to hers, she knew that Christ died for this man, and she forced herself to reach to him. As she took his hand, she felt the power of God come and melt the hatred at that very moment.

I pray for you to ask God at this moment, to give you forgiveness for any moment as memories that may need your release. As certain persons or situations come to mind, I pray for His courage to become yours, now and here with your Savior who has experienced hate, betrayal, and abuse like no one on this earth.

A journal and prayer section on this chapter can be found on page 97.

# 9

# WHAT IS THE STRONGEST, WISEST INFLUENCE?

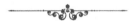

*Thousands of diseases were cured as Jesus walked on the earth. He knew the steps to take to enter each village, to find and heal the lost sheep. He knows the whys and hows of the brain. He knew the demoniac's behavior was not of this world and neither denied it nor gave it special attention.*

THE LORD KNOWS the purpose for every child. There are children whose bodies have, in some ways, become prisons for their existence.

God understands what it means to be imprisoned. He had times of action, speaking, and silence. Perhaps you are now in one of those times.

Misunderstanding has caused terrible suffering in the past. There was a time when Greek physicians categorized any unexplainable behavior as a divine disease. These ranged from strange or unpredictable actions or speech to convulsions. In the 1950's and 1960's, there was a general agreement that strange, repetitive behavior was a form of psychosis. Today many physicians have labels for many of the divine diseases, but it is rare that they go beyond treating the symptoms to finding a cure.

During the pre-Christian era, children were taken to healers. During Greek and Roman times, such children were occasionally sewed into the wet skin of a goat to calm such behaviors. Healers often failed, with many children never making it through "treatment," which commonly included rejection or mistreatment due to superstition.

Families would be turned out of their homes and villages because of fear and lack of understanding. Children also died if the village healer demanded torture or abandonment. With the Industrial Revolution, a new value was put on children—money. Even mild behavior deviations were dealt with physically and severely. Today, there are laws to prevent children becoming a commodity, and severe physical punishment is frowned upon. Wrong attitudes, superstition, and abandonment are still present.

Spiritually, we live in a time when divine diseases are often misunderstood because even though we have advanced in our technology, our accumulation of knowledge have left parents with many hundreds of avenues to pursue. Intelligence and reason have made finding the path confusing to traverse.

But we have one who answers prayers and can guide us in the decisions we make.

We relocated from Utah to Montana in 2000, and I began working with Christian at home one-on-one.

One particular morning, I heard a full, clear sentence spoken from Christian's bedroom. He was four years old, but had not spoken more than two numbers or letters in a phrase.

I heard, "Mommy, mommy, I have to tell you about my dream!"

As I pushed the door open, I saw my little man sitting up, looking at me. The first thing I noticed as I walked toward him was the pupils of his eyes.

Until that moment, his eyes remained dilated most of the time; he had extremely slow pupillary response. His pupils looked normal, and his hazel eyes were full of excitement as he started describing his dream.

Christian reached up and put his hands on both of my cheeks and looked into my eyes. He said, "Jesus put His hands on my face and said, 'Christian, you don't have to face those demons anymore.'"

I held him for a long, long time. He had drawn pictures of his nightmares and woke up screaming many nights. He continued to tell me that the monsters were all around him when Jesus came - and they scattered.

I felt God's presence that morning—like a mist; a tangible presence and there was joy wrapped all around us.

# 10

# The Maze of Theory

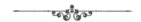

## What Is a Diagnosis?

> We need to be very careful not to view the snapshot as an end-all. Every one of us have made mistakes, had bad days, and traumatic experiences where fear or rejection took hold. If in the midst of this we took only that snapshot to determine the function and success and happiness for the rest of our lives, it would be very shallow and a limiting view of the future.

A DIAGNOSIS IS a "snapshot" of a child's behavior or function. It shows by one measure or another the level of function in a child's auditory, sensory, visual, cognitive, speech, physical, emotional, psychological, or intellectual functions.

After Christian's dream, his pupils constricted easier and administering the neurodevelopment exercises was much easier. Before the dream, he could repeat only two numbers or letters back when asked. He had been delayed in the reflexive/expressive areas of the brain.

Each of us are developing in our relationship with God, as spiritual beings having a physical experience through the auditory, visual and sensory areas of life. Problems with perspective, understanding, and maturing in faith are levels of "function" we see in one another.

Christian's vocabulary had been purely a recording, saying phonetically difficult words with no association to what the words meant. Social interactions were difficult and being hypersensitive to sound caused problems whenever there were alarms, loud music, crowds and even church worship services. Midrange tones would cause him to cover his ears, scream, hide and cry. He wasn't able to filter or mix sounds to acceptable levels.

As a result of the differences of opinion as to the causes of problems, different explanations, discernments, and treatment approaches are devised. I found the following popular explanations were guiding much of the counseling I received from well-trained and well meaning people and specialists:

1. All problems are caused by psychological factors, and so we can ignore organic or physical causes.

2. All problems are physical in some way, and the behavior is the result.

Some of the current available treatments include negative/positive conditioning or behavioral therapy, educational approaches, special schools/training, and modification through diet or intake of vitamins. Purpose and potential are a gift of God and based on relationship rather than rules. No single approach has been the answer for all children, and most parents acquire services in many different modalities of treatment to find the unique sequence to unlock their child's function and potential.

Within six months of exercises and Linda Kane's encouragement, Christian's processing had accelerated to that of a six-year-old's and language was developing. At first he was stuttering terribly and had many reversals in both speech and writing. I was encouraged to focus on the development of his language center/dominant hemisphere, which took a few more months. His reversals and stuttering completely disappeared! He was reading second-grade level books aloud by the end of the year!

Samonas sound therapy also brought changes to how he handled loud environments, and in time he no longer had to cover his ears for loud sounds. Today he plays music and leads worship without opposition to volume.

When we started with exercises, Christian was exhibiting echolalia—the immediate or delayed echoing or repetition of whole, unanalyzed expressions and sounds. He could repeat a sound like a recording, but without understanding.

Christian could show me where loud electrical noise was coming from and replay musical tones more than anything else. In time I understood that he was hearing those sounds/tones with more intensity than verbal tones—which explained by months of speech therapy had not achieved what we had hoped.

Part of Christian's rehabilitation included removing musical tones for a time while working to establish language. His auditory system needed to be "taught" all the sounds needed for language, or like most children on the autism spectrum who play music, he would replay, but not create music. While removing musical tones, we input language and worked on filtering, memory and cognition.

When we reintroduced instruments and his keyboard several months later, Christian began composing original orchestra pieces.

Many parents understand that there are multiple intelligences and learning styles and observe their child's strengths so they can adjust teaching methods. If a child does not learn as quickly while sitting, we may teach the spelling words while they go up and down the stairs.

When damage, trauma or injustice occurs, it is similar to cellular development in the brain creating a delay. We can ask God to heal the unseen. Ninety-nine percent of all protection, provision and intervention happens in His sight, not ours.

As I worked with Christian, because of sensory and mobility issues, I had to perform each exercise with him - arm/hand to his arm/hand, crawling, creeping on the floor, wearing eye patches and ear plugs. What I experienced was healing for my own neural damage as I came alongside my son. My auditory processing/memory was totally changed and analytical processes, communication and organization made it possible for me to study neurodevelopment.

I would have coped with low processing and difficulties for the rest of my life, but God provided a path to restoration. Another hidden treasure on this road less traveled.

# 11

# Unlocking Your Child's Potential Is a Journey Not a Destination

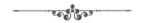

*There is more to the puzzle. We have to unlock not just sensory conditions, but emotional and spiritual issues blocking wholeness.*

Without a spiritual foundation (believing in unseen help), the nervous system is an impossible and complex map to navigate. Finding the correct visual, auditory, or tactile sensory diet is as important as nutrition. Without it, the brain and central nervous system will not be satisfied; and behaviors, which are function problems in the underlying areas of the brain, will continue. Some examples are the following:

- intolerance of textures
- sensitivities to smells

- auditory sensitivity (talking too loud, playing music too loud)
- auditory or visual processing
- short-term and long-term memory problems
- speech problems
- tonal problems
- balance problems
- reflex aberrations
- hyperactivity
- poor manual competence
- sensory distortions
- attention aberrations
- significant learning disability

There are distractions, emotional issues, and unseen foundational areas in the brain causing perceptual problems. Addictions, learning problems, and aberrant behavior are now considered common, but I believe we suffer from a type of spiritual autism as well. Fears, abuse, neglect, memories and addictions are complex and these may distort our perceptions and challenge our relationships and beliefs.

Ethologists believe that space and territory acquisitions are basic needs; space and territory are measurable and stable, predictable for normal brains. Unknown things in the environment or space can impose uncomfortable sights, sounds, or feelings that cannot be controlled.

For the person with hindrances, addictions, missing relationships or disobedience, they may not be seeing, hearing or sensing right and wrong.

The only foundation strong enough to endure the struggles of this life in our relationship with our children is our relationship with our Creator. Our purpose in worshipping Him is to find the purpose that child is to fulfill on this earth.

Even in the maze of sensory, auditory and visual learning styles, multiple intelligences, and learning problems and disabilities, we can grow in character, prayer, and faith. Unlocking our own potential and that of our child's is a lifelong pursuit, not a destination.

No one who knows Christian suspects the difficulties he faced. I remember thinking he must be a David or Joseph for such a tremendous amount of difficulty to happen at so young an age. Like David, he has written many original compositions and desires to follow his dreams to play music and tell the story of God's miracle in his life.

# 12

# ACCEL-ACADEMY CONCLUSION

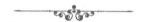

## To Unlimited and Beyond

*The most important question I would ask is this:
Are you willing to do whatever it takes,
make whatever adjustment,
to help yourself or your child?*

WHEN I LEARNED to ride a motorcycle, I was told to look beyond the turn—to where I was going. What this meant was, if I looked to my feet instead of ahead, I would automatically turn too quickly or lean too far. I watched another new rider tip over during a turn on the safety range. Focus determines reality—I have to focus up ahead, where I plan to go, rather than on the cracks, potholes, and problems of the moment. Otherwise, I could easily end up on the ground.

He turned and said, "How about 'In Good Hands' for the name? I wrote the title and he took the paper to the judges. He played beautifully and spoke to the judges about his story.

As we returned home, our vehicle slid off the road when we hit black ice. The car flipped several times, but we had minor injuries. There were twelve accidents on the same stretch of road, and we were one of the few families to walk away from an accident.

I pray that your vision will soar above every *unlikely* event to the *unlimited future* God has for you and your children!

Christian and I offer Accel-Academy courses to explain the basics of neurodevelopment and teach exercises that create opportunities to improve memory and so much more! See http://stephslc.wix.com/learningsuccess for more information.

christianmichaelunlimited
@gmail.com

# A Debriefing of the Neurodevelopmental Approach

THE FOLLOWING INFORMATION will point you to research articles, seminars, and opportunities to learn more.

The neurodevelopmental approach is a method of accelerating learning and development for those anywhere on the spectrum of loss of function. The exercises relate specifically to underlying areas of the brain such behaviors and functions as attention; focus; auditory and visual precision; short- and long-term memory; filtering; hypo- and hypersensitivities to auditory, visual, or tactile stimuli; metabolic issues and compliance; and addressing the foundation that is known to specifically change the way the whole system receives, processes, stores, and responds to various stimuli.

The goal is to have the whole child or adult be able to process sensory information (visual, auditory, tactile input, and functional output) by creating an excellent foundation that will affect every area of academics, emotions, communication, and physical responses. In this successful state, it will be easier to unlock potential for the appropriate emotional and academic responses to stimuli received in any environment with permanent results.

The science that is the basis of the treatment needs to be considered if we want to achieve permanent results rather than cope with behaviors permanently. The solution is not better building materials (therapies) but the foundation that holds up the materials.

The ND approach is special in that it helps more areas that you can observe. Although the brain and central nervous system are hidden, they manage every aspect of life—from tasting, to smelling foul foods, hearing and filtering the sounds of vehicles passing outside, cooking, and cleaning—processing millions of pieces of sensory information while directing our lungs, heart, and kidneys to work out their life-giving tasks. They are part of the blueprint we don't even glimpse unless there is something that stops working.

The methods we use are modification of the system itself. Input and exercises directed at the foundation of the brain and the auditory, visual, or tactile system that is receiving, processing, storing, and responding. The brain develops in a very specific order, so the areas of development are addressed in the same order. The three paths we use to bring information to the foundation of the brain are the auditory, visual, and tactile systems.

Each area of the brain must be developed prior to moving on to the next area. The neurodevelopmental profile shows the input and output functions that correspond with the areas of the brain starting with the pons, medulla, midbrain, and up to the higher cortex. Once we identify what level the brain is developed to, we teach the specific exercises that will stimulate that area of the brain. We also teach the frequency, intensity, and duration that the stimulation will need to be applied to modify each of the specific systems at the area of development. They are connected like a chain, so we focus on the level of development of the auditory, visual, and tactile system in the brain rather than one system receiving stimulation (visual) while others are left alone.

The neurodevelopmental approach is designed for children who have been diagnosed with a variety of labels from mild (learning delays, ADD) to severe (brain injuries, autism, strokes.) To begin, a child is evaluated then the parents, families, teachers, and specialists are taught to observe and respond specifically to the underlying brain issues of the diagnosis, disease, or injury. Function is accelerated when persons provide the nervous system a minimum of ten weeks to three months of specific, targeted stimulation then this is reevaluated and continued for the remainder of the year. The brain will require the stimulation be provided specifically at the correct frequency and duration to create change.

I began the restorative part of our journey with my son with the resources available at a conference meeting Linda Kane, an ICAN Neurodevelopmentalist. She has written a book that describes the NeuroDevelopmental Approach, which is available for purchase at www.hope-future.org/store/c1/Featured_Products.html.

Additional resources and visual evaluations are available through another partner site at www.littlegiantsteps.com/services. Begin learning how to unlock God's purpose and development in your children today!

The treatment and results of neurodevelopment have been replicated by a wide variety of specialists working with a wide variety of children since 1959. Hope and a Future is one branch within the International Christian Association of Neurodevelopmentalists, who have branches in many cities in the United States.

# Study and Prayer Guide Quotes, Meditations, Journals, and Prayers

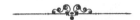

The points on this map of unlikely places do not determine your future.

# 1

# FROM UNLIKELY PLACES

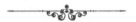

EVERY PERSON IN my life has faced difficulty, fear, trauma, or abuse. It is comforting but also sobering to know that every person I meet has been or is in some sort of trial.

In recovering, the first step is to admit that we are powerless and that our lives are unmanageable. Maybe you are in a place right now where hope has fled and there is no vision for what is up ahead. I was in that place—a most unlikely circumstance encountering severe problems with my son Christian's tactility, speech, and vision, when there were unlikely possibilities. I was desperate to find answers, and maybe you are also.

Your future will depend on accepting moments of truth here and now that will begin creating opportunities for adjustment, healing, and hope for your future. Desperation can be the doorway to unlikely creativity and courage.

My life quote is this: "I know the plans I have for you, plans to prosper you and not to harm you. Plans to give you hope and a future." Many have memorized this and written about this quote, read in the story, "Jeremiah's Letter to the Captives."

Now these are the words of the letter that Jeremiah the prophet sent from Jerusalem to the remainder of the elders who were carried away captive—to the priests, the prophets, and all the people whom Nebuchadnezzar had carried away captive from Jerusalem to Babylon.

I don't need to describe the emotions of a family raising a child with disabilities in any more certain terms than this. Captive. From the moment of waking to the sometimes remote hours of sleeping or sleeplessness, it feels like we are living without the right to our own lives. To begin, let us define *we*—the people in your life, family, and experience:

1. _____

2. _____

3. _____

4. _____

5. _____

6. _____

7. _____

8. _____

One of the most difficult steps in the journey is when expectations were changed. Because this wasn't in our control, there is a painful process of discovering, rather than planning what comes ahead.

Take a moment to list your personal expectations and emotions that you have struggled with in this journey.

1. _____
2. _____
3. _____
4. _____
5. _____
6. _____
7. _____
8. _____
9. _____
10. _____

God is very close to us during every moment, every step. God meets us here in this unlikely place with a promise: God draws near to the brokenhearted. Take each of the names and each of the expectations verbally to God in prayer.

> Lord, I pray that you meet each (name each person _____) at this moment. I give you these expectations and emotions that

I have been struggling with (name each one
_____). Where the unknown
has released fear, anger, and hopelessness, show us
that You hold the future in Your hands and You will
not leave us for the duration of this journey. Let this
unlikely place be the defining moment for belief,
courage, and healing. In Jesus's name. Amen.

While providing passive exercises to my autistic son,
which he did not accept, agree, or cooperate with, I came
to realize that instruction, guidance, and opportunities are
passive input in our lives. When facing difficulties, I will
open my Bible and study the words and situations such
as Psalms. I write out the words in my journal, or if the
situation is especially difficult, I carry the words, written on
note cards. During emotional times, the analytic part of our
thinking is disengaged. Holding the truth in front of me is
my spiritual remedy, which I see as more important than
taking vitamin C for a cold.

# 2

# Unlikely Courage

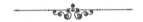

*In our journey, there are opportunities for
development. Potential exists for growth in every
situation, but the way we interact with those
situations is through physical sense and emotion.
We tend to separate our mind, will, and emotions
from our physical experience, but there is a link
between what happens in this world and how it
affects the unseen and the eternal.*

The miracle of the brain is its ability to respond to new stimulation. Creating the opportunity at the specific level we need at the precise time for the proper length at the right intensity is another aspect of God's ability to meet us right where we are.

God gives us access to wisdom for every situation and area that is in need of the release of answers, resources, or courage. We come to believe that a power greater than ourselves can restore us, which gives meaning and purpose to our lives. When we define success for ourselves, we cannot forget the unseen spiritual reality that is developing in us, through us, and around us.

There is a God that can restore us!

List any developmental issues you are aware of, known incidents, or issues that would affect development. Try and determine which part of the nervous system is the most affected (auditory, visual, taste/smell, tactile deep pressure, or light touch).

1. _____
2. _____
3. _____
4. _____
5. _____
6. _____
7. _____
8. _____
9. _____
10. _____

Lord, I ask that I will see beyond the current issues. I bring to you each physical (name area_____) that has affected my child or myself. I want to accept that change is now possible and that you have power greater than anything I have trusted in. Intervene in each of the physical, emotional, and spiritual areas that are a concern, in Jesus's name.

# 3

# Unlikely Clarity

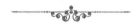

> How one views the nature of God impacts how
> one views anything that occurs in his world.

Jeremiah was a prophet who lived under the command not to marry or have children to illustrate his message that judgment was pending. The next generation would be swept away, and salvation could not be divorced from faith in God and a right covenantal relationship expressed by obedience.

Having a child with special needs causes us to slow down and see priorities differently. We need time spent focusing intentionally on faith or we automatically respond with emotion, fear, associations or triggers.

1. _____
2. _____
3. _____
4. _____

5. _____

6. _____

7. _____

8. _____

9. _____

10. _____

In Jeremiah's day, the rulers had led the people astray. Models of therapy, diagnosis, advice, or counsel can be similar to the rulers, priests, or false prophets. Although many methods are very popular and effective at some level, there is a limit in unlocking the potential of the whole person. Have you ever tried a specific therapy or technique to modify behaviors and were unable to get the results that you believed you could get and ultimately questioned why it was not working, that something just didn't feel right?

Having a child with special needs causes us to slow down and see priorities differently. We are dependent, and we need time spent in God's truth every day or we forget what truth is. We need time to pray and to share with others our hopes, growth, and truth.

In the midst of seeming captivity, we have to understand that there is no other foundation or relationship that can help or save our children. We don't understand what caused the situation, but today, this moment, we know we have a choice. Those who listened to the truth were saved in

Jeremiah's day. The situation for those who remained in the city and would not heed or obey was destruction. When I was told Christian would be institutionalized for life, I had a choice—to become angry and turn away from God, or believe He was good regardless of what happened. To continue to choose to find healthy and truthful people to spend time with and find activities and fellowship that would help me live in truth.

> Lord, you know the truth in every circumstance. I ask that You silence all confusion and contend with all influences that are contending with Your truth and path for my life and that of my child. I ask that You be our guide. In Jesus's name. Amen.

# 4

# Unlikely Purpose and Wholeness

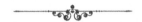

Every child can reach his or her purpose in God.

THERE ARE UNDERLYING nerve brain inputs, outputs, and function that we can observe. List any areas of the sensory system that are now apparent (grunting, banging, swinging, tics, verbal slurs, pain tolerance or intolerance, textures, smells, or diet).

1. _____
2. _____
3. _____
4. _____
5. _____
6. _____
7. _____

8. _____

9. _____

10. _____

As you observe the list, is there a specific area that stands out? Banging or noise would indicate auditory system; looking out of the peripheral vision or sitting too close to the TV indicates the visual system.

1. _____

2. _____

3. _____

4. _____

5. _____

Other hindrances to our development are more complex like DNA strands, generational destructive cycles, word curses, abuse, and emotional wounds that have misdirected our responses and kept us and our children from wholeness.

List any known destructive cycles, emotional behaviors such as outbursts, specific abuse, or issues your family generations have experienced.

1. _____

2. _____

3. _____

4. _____

5. _____

6. _____

7. _____

8. _____

9. _____

10. _____

God, we know that you see what needs intervention. You made a tremendous sacrifice to make change now and here. The blood of Jesus is all powerful to restore damage and function and stop cycles that are hindering development. I thank You for purchasing my life and the life of my child, for Your purposes. In Jesus' name. Amen.

# 5

# Unlikely Involvement

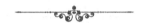

*Similar to a military landing on an occupied island, there is chaos when God steps in.*

God had a specific order for my home, my budget, and my time. I had to be intentional about activities, the atmosphere, and events of our lives during recovery. We choose how we spend the 86,400 seconds we have been given each day. Just as what we put in our mouths will affect physical development, how we spend our time will affect the foundation of physiological, spiritual, and emotional development our children experience.

Think about and list daily activities.

1. _____
2. _____
3. _____
4. _____

5. _____

6. _____

7. _____

8. _____

9. _____

10. _____

Look for any activities that may be exchanged in the future for quiet time or changes to the sensory diet (less visual, more auditory or interaction) when with your child.

1. _____

2. _____

3. _____

4. _____

5. _____

Look for any variables that may be exchanged in the future—such as buying audiobooks instead of visual/ movies or computer games.

1. _____

2. _____

3. _____

4. _____

5. _____

When God gave me the opportunity to raise a special child, He was giving me a merciful choice that, if I accepted, would change my heart. When I said yes to motherhood, I was able to relive in childhood with Christian. There were also a few unique problems that would change not just my heart but my self-interest, devotion, and especially my prayers.

> Let's pray: I thank You, Lord, for having intentional order in creation. You also have intentional order for my priorities in life. Please rearrange any therapy sessions, activities, and budget that I may begin not to live reactively to whatever comes along, but receive the best You have for this life—inside and out. In Jesus' name, Amen.

# 6

# WHAT IS ABNORMAL BEHAVIOR?

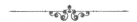

Truth and wisdom are what exists after man's opinions disappear.

I BELIEVE THAT through Christ, adults and children will have a better opportunity to develop beyond the trauma and labels of the past, but we have to look beyond the labels and behaviors to the foundation.

The fear of the Lord is the beginning of wisdom, truth, and freedom for every man, woman, and child. Make a list and write in desired responses and attitudes.

1. _____
2. _____
3. _____
4. _____
5. _____

6. _____

7. _____

8. _____

9. _____

10. _____

The atmosphere, culture, and environment we live in affect how we recognize or respond negatively or positively to truth. Our background and experience cause us to form opinions, but truth exists is unchangeable.

> Lord, now and here, Your love covers a multitude of attitudes, behaviors, and every unknown. I pray now to break these cycles and behaviors. Help me to turn to you first, in Jesus's name. Amen.

# 7

# Unlikely Building Material—Day after Day

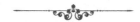

*Practical day-to-day activities are part of the journey, part of learning about faith.*

BACK TO OUR story with Jeremiah, the Bible says, "Build houses and dwell in them; plant gardens and eat their fruit. Take wives and beget sons and daughters; and take wives for your sons and give daughters to husbands, so that they may bear sons and daughters—that you may be increased there, and not diminished" (Jeremiah 29:5–6, New King James Version).

Jeremiah gave the captives direction for their practical lives. Continue to prepare for the future, continue to increase and live. Build houses and dwell in them; plant gardens and eat their fruit. Continue to betroth your children and plan for their futures. We still sleep and eat and budget and walk, but there is more—do not let the devil diminish your hope. Your lives will be much simpler focusing on the practical things of life, building and planting, but your lives are to increase and not diminish. That only happens when you fix your eyes beyond the cracks in the sidewalk of the present situation. Hope is the key to the future—fixing your eyes on what is unseen, not what is seen.

Acts 17:26 says that "He has made from one blood every nation of men to dwell on all the face of the earth, and has determined their pre-appointed times and the boundaries of their dwellings."

Acts 17:26 says that He determined your time and dwelling. Right now, right here.

Acts 17:27–28 says, "So that they should seek the Lord, in the hope that they might grope for Him and find Him, though He is not far from each one of us; for in Him we live and move and have our being."

He has been seeking you to find and save you. Life is about finding the most important. Salvation is a glimpse of God, of eternity. Though He is not far from each one of us, we can live years on this earth without seeking Him.

He paid a purchase price for your exile, that you would have your life, your day-to-day in Him. He knows where you are and how many appointments and doctors and tests and labels this world will place.

When Linda Kane first described to me how each one of Christian's function issues could be addressed, I was overwhelmed with hope and knew that my prayers were being answered.

Lord, You know how the practical things fit like puzzle pieces into the mysterious puzzle of life and development. I acknowledge that You have appointed the boundaries and times of deliverance. My heart needs to be lifted so I can set my hands to build and arms to plant and my heart to hope again. Break all hope deferred and despair. Remove all unbelief in Jesus' name. I ask for joy and strength to arise now. I ask that I may know Your voice and Your ways from this day and believe!

# 8

# Unlikely Inventory

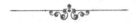

> The brain stores information, not like a photo
> album that can be closed at will, but more like an
> open gallery that places photographs in moments
> by association.

Truth is like a new language to most of us. It will take time, but we need to cultivate a relationship with Him that is not casual but intentional. Many people are led astray because they do not know what voice or truth to listen to. There have been false prophets in every area of society and every decade of history. The Bible says, "If the foundations are destroyed, what can the righteous do?" (Psalm 11:3, New King James Version).

Back to our story with Jeremiah, the Bible says, "And seek the peace of the city where I have caused you to be carried away captive, and pray to the Lord for it; for in its peace you will have peace" (Jeremiah 29:7, New King James Version). In the midst of captivity a totally new concept is included in this letter. They were to pray for the well-being of their captors. A special inventory of our past, our history, and our present dwelling can reveal places in our thinking where we hold ourselves, other people, places, or situations responsible.

Our obedience requires a supernatural strength that only comes from Christ. The One Who Forgives gave Corrie Ten Boom the strength as she silently warred, prayed, and asked for the means to forgive. She states that as he extended his hand to hers, she knew that Christ died for this man, and she forced herself to reach to him. As she took his hand, she felt the power of God come and melt the hatred at that very moment.

Make a list of all persons we have harmed and become willing to make amends; make a list of all persons who have harmed us and become willing to forgive.

We may have more situations or persons that need amends or our forgiveness. I pray that God will give you forgiveness for any moment as memories that may need your release. As certain persons or situations come to mind, I pray for His courage to become yours here and now with your Savior who has experienced hate, betrayal, and abuse like no one on this earth. He sees and knows this moment and is here to release strength in your obedience to Him.

1. _____

2. _____

3. _____

4. _____

5. _____

> I come before you, Lord, in Jesus's mighty name asking for your revelation of any area where there is unforgiveness. I recognize the pain and trauma have created a snapshot with _____ (person or place) that I need to release. I want forgiveness as you have given as an act of my will, in obedience to Your desire—that I may be no longer tormented by evil thoughts, emotions, or hatred. In Jesus's name, Amen.

Take as much time as you need for this step. I encourage fasting (can be food, activities, or media). If there is a need, make direct amends wherever possible except when to do so would injure them or others. This is a time of release. You may need to write a letter, or put a chair in front of you and talk as if the person is sitting there with you—especially if the person is no longer alive. This is also a good time to share this with a person you trust.

The journey of recovery continues with taking daily time to release those who wrong us, and when wrong, promptly admit it. When wronged, promptly forgive.

# 9

# WHAT IS THE STRONGEST, WISEST INFLUENCE?

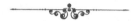

*Thousands of diseases were cured as Jesus walked on the earth. He knew the steps to take to enter each village, to find and heal the lost sheep. He knows the whys and hows of the brain. He knew the demoniac's behavior was not of this world and neither denied it nor gave it special attention.*

THE LORD KNOWS the purpose for every child.

God understands what it means to be imprisoned. He had times of action, speaking, and silence. Perhaps you are now in one of those times. There is hope. There are so many seasons where we may feel misunderstood or confused.

Years ago I read *Tortured for Christ* by Richard Wurmbrand, who courageously resisted the communists' control of the church and went underground. He and his wife both went to prison, and he suffered torture at the hands of those who misunderstood. I continue today to advocate for those persecuted for their faith, knowing many of our brothers and sisters in Christ have witnessed the death, torture, or imprisonment of family members where individuals or governments have decided to wipe out Christianity. I choose to read and pray daily for these precious ones, knowing that faith has *unlimited* vision and looks beyond the present situation into eternity. They persevere because their eyes are focused to eternity and beyond.

"Now faith is the substance of things hoped for, the evidence of things not seen. For by it the elders obtained a good testimony. By faith we understand that the worlds were framed by the word of God, so that the things which are seen were not made of things which are visible" (Hebrews 11:1–3, *New King James Version).*

> Let us pray: Lord, today there are many directions and voices claiming they are the way. Healers may fail, and misunderstanding is still present, but You do not fail. You are the Way, the Truth, and the Life. I ask that You give me vision in my journey of faith and practical discernment in the therapy I am to pursue for my child. I ask that You navigate each time I feel the waves of misunderstanding, knowing that what touches us, touches You. In Jesus's name. Amen.

# 10

# THE MAZE OF THEORY

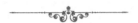

## What Is a Diagnosis?

*We need to be very careful not to view the snapshot as an end-all. Every one of us has made mistakes, had bad days, and traumatic experiences where fear or rejection took hold. If in the midst of this we took only that snapshot to determine the function and success and happiness for the rest of our lives, it would be very shallow and limiting view of the future.*

A DIAGNOSIS IS a "snapshot" of a child's behavior or function. It shows by one measure or another the level of function in a child's auditory, sensory, visual, cognitive, speech, physical, emotional, psychological or intellectual functions.

If we use a snapshot of the behavior and understand it is only a symptom of an underlying cause, then we will focus beyond intervention to the foundation. What we choose will affect potential and function both in the present and future.

List the current treatments or teaching methods now present in the life of your child (learning styles, kinesthetic therapy, speech therapy, occupational therapy, diet, etc.).

1. _____

2. _____

3. _____

4. _____

5. _____

6. _____

7. _____

8. _____

Lord, every parent you have entrusted with life needs your wisdom. Show us what tactile, auditory, and visual strengths and weaknesses are not present. You already know how to unlock the potential in every person. Confirm what intervention or treatment is needed to create a successful learning environment, and remove what is unessential in Jesus' name. Amen.

# 11

# Unlocking Your Child's Potential Is a Journey Not a Destination

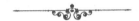

*There is more to the puzzle. We have to unlock not just sensory conditions, but emotional and spiritual issues blocking wholeness.*

There are many neurological problems that need to be addressed with a spiritual foundation in focus.

Many behaviors have function problems in the underlying areas of the brain: lack of coordination, developmental delay, strabismus, laterality dysfunctions, toe walking, scoliosis, balance problems, reflex aberrations, hyperactivity, poor manual competence, sensory distortions, attention aberrations, and significant learning disability. Spiritual hindrances to growth have underlying areas of dysfunction that are complex and personal to each person—fears, experiences, abuse, neglect, memories, and perception.

Daily we can use tools to move past those hindrances. Daily we seek through prayer and meditation to improve our conscious contact with God, praying only for knowledge of his will for us and the power to carry that out.

Write out your prayer here:

_____
_____
_____
_____
_____
_____
_____
_____
_____
_____
_____

# 12

# Accel-Academy Conclusion

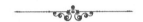

## To Unlimited and Beyond

*The most important question I would ask is this: Are you willing to do whatever it takes, make whatever adjustment, to help yourself or your child?*

DAILY MEDITATION, INVENTORY, prayer, and evaluation of time, relationships, and activities are gifts that keep my mind healthy and my spiritual life moving forward.

God's plans are to prosper you, and not to harm you; He plans to give you hope and a future!

May you use these tools daily for the rest of your life.

May your life be transformed by prayer and meditation.

May your sight come into sharp, faith-focused vision as you prepare for the future God has for you and your children! From unlikely to unlimited and beyond!

Christian and I offer Accel-Academy day-training that gives an overview of neurodevelopment. For more information, please visit: stephslc.wix.com/learningsuccess

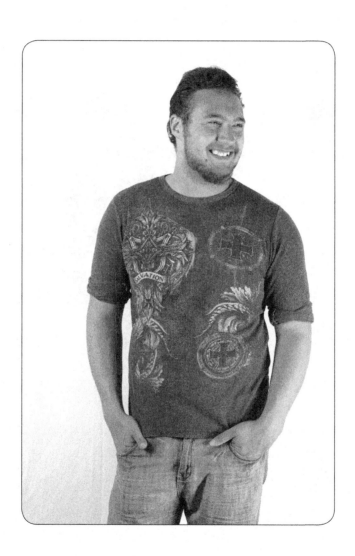

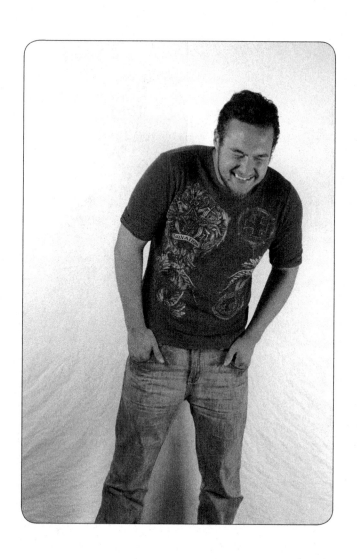

**Desired Change: Attending/Compliance**
PROGRESS TOWARD DESIRED CHANGE: (S) Christian is currently attending on level IA at step C2d at 100%. Christian had an average of 74% General, 47% Please and 15% Need with 21 directions not followed for the month. Behaviors are monitored daily. Christian had 54 physical aggressions to person, 19 physical aggressions toward objects and 9 bites to others during this month. (I) Christian is receiving directions using the general precision command format. The attending program is utilized to increase attending skills. A token system is in place to address all physical aggressions. (P) Continue using the precision command format to monitor compliance daily. Continue probing Christian through level IA of the attending program. Continue use of the token system, and consider alternate reinforcers for appropriate behaviors.

**Desired Change: Language/Cognition**
PROGRESS TOWARD DESIRED CHANGE: (S) Christian is currently probing through Level IA of the attending hierarchy. He has completed C2c with 100% attending. Christian is verbalizing for all wants and needs. (I) Christian is reinforced when he verbalized his needs and wants appropriately. (P) Continue probing Christian through the core attending program and begin Level IIA using 5-step programs--object imitation, motor imitation, matching etc.

**Desired Change: Parental Involvement**
PROGRESS TOWARDS DESIRED CHANGE: (S) Parents have daily contact through home notes and notebook. Christian's mother comes into the classroom on Wednesday afternoons. (I) Staff utilizes daily home notes, telephone contact etc as needed. (P) Continue use of daily home notes to parents, telephone contact and scheduling parent in the classroom.

**Desired Change: Social/Self-Help**
PROGRESS TOWARDS DESIRED CHANGE: (S) Christian participates in all group activities such as calendar, free-choice, snack, computer, story and song. Christian actively seeks other children to play with him. Christian toilets independently. (I) Christian is reinforced for appropriate social interactions. Prompting, shaping and fading techniques are utilized to increase Christians self-help skills. DRO is utilized in all group sessions. (P) Continue reinforcing Christians appropriate social interactions. DRO and other techniques.

_____
Supervisor's Signature/Title (if necessary)

_____
Therapist's Signature/Title

VALLEY MENTAL HEALTH
SDS GROUP MONTHLY SUMMARY

Patient Name _Christian Tuiplotu_
Patient I.D.# _084a1700_
Month _September_  Year _1999_
Unit _4/1_

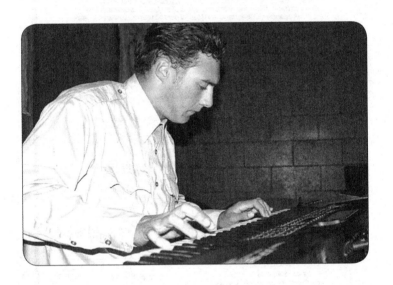

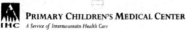

**PRIMARY CHILDREN'S MEDICAL CENTER**
IHC  *A Service of Intermountain Health Care*

100 North Medical Drive
Salt Lake City, Utah 84113
(801) 588-2000
(801) 588-2460 Fax

**REHAB WEST, 3845 West 4700 South, Suite 102, Taylorsville, Utah 84118**
**(801)964-4060**

June 9, 1999

RE: Chrisitan Tuipulotu
DOB: 1/10/95
ID#: 529-41-2007

To Whom It May Concenr:

Christian is a 4 year old who was referred for an occupational therapy evaluation by Dr. Rober Lillard, for concerns with sensory processing issues. He is diagnosed with Pervasive Developmental Disorder and Oppositional-Defiant Behavior. He was seen for an evaluation at Primary Children's Rehab West on 4/29/99. During this evaluation, Christian demonstrated difficulty with many sensory processing issues which could affect his functional performance in daily tasks. Christian has difficulty processing the various sensory information in his environment. He demonstrates difficulty with his tactile system as seen by hypersensitivity to various tactile situations which make interacting with peers difficult for him. He also shows signs of difficulty with hypersensitivity to auditory input. Christian has many behaviors seeking vestibular and proprioceptive input. His sensory processing difficulties, especially related to modulation, affect his attention and ability to learn new skills in all areas.

Occupational therapy is recommended to address the sensory processing issues to assist Christian with normalizing his responses to various sensory input, improve regulation of behaviors which will assist him with his attention and interaction in social skills for age, ability to learn new functional fine motor and self-help skills. Please authorize weekly sixty minute occupational therapy session for six months.

Thank you for your consideration of this matter. If you have any additional questions or concerns please contact this Center at (801)964-4060.

Sincerely,

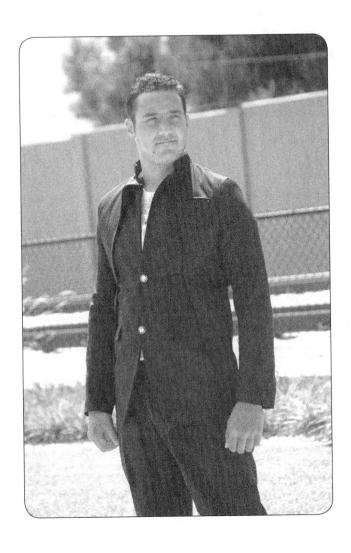

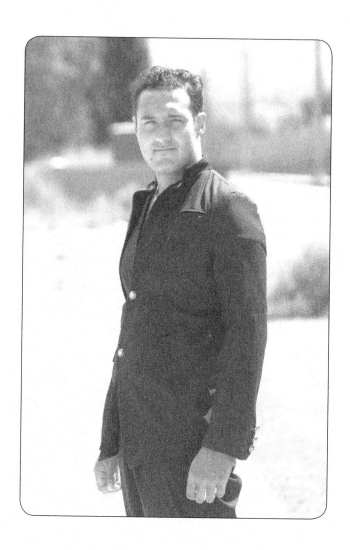

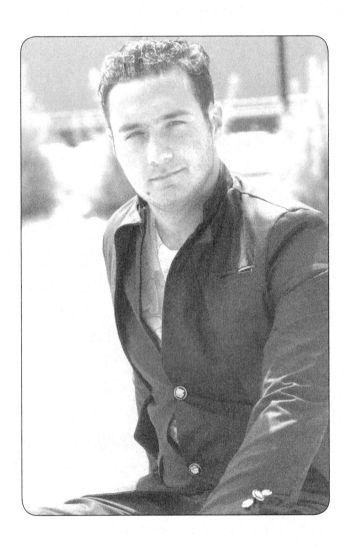

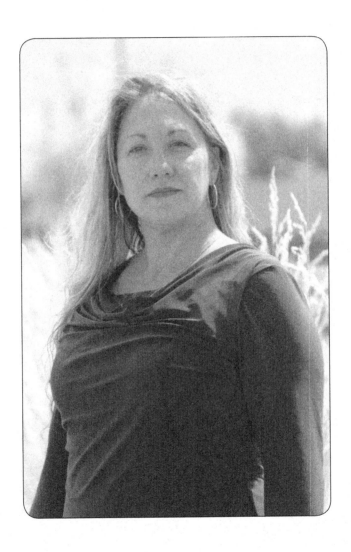

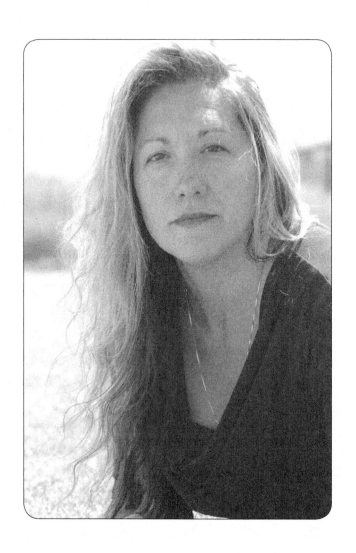

# listen|imagine|view|experience

AUDIO BOOK DOWNLOAD INCLUDED WITH THIS BOOK!

In your hands you hold a complete digital entertainment package. In addition to the paper version, you receive a free download of the audio version of this book. Simply use the code listed below when visiting our website. Once downloaded to your computer, you can listen to the book through your computer's speakers, burn it to an audio CD or save the file to your portable music device (such as Apple's popular iPod) and listen on the go!

How to get your free audio book digital download:

1. Visit www.tatepublishing.com and click on the e|LIVE logo on the home page.
2. Enter the following coupon code:
   9072-af69-becb-86a7-8879-bd3f-9f05-9cef
3. Download the audio book from your e|LIVE digital locker and begin enjoying your new digital entertainment package today!